MICRODOSING CANNABIS EVOLUTION

Table of Contents

[What is Microdosing?](#)
[History of Microdosing](#)
[What Does CBD Feel Like?](#)
[Microdosing CBD for Beginners](#)
[Microdosing And Me: A Useful (And Honest) Guide To CBD And Pain](#)
[7 Benefits and Uses of CBD Oil (Plus Side Effects)](#)

What is Microdosing?

Microdosing CBD is a technique that involves taking very small amounts of cannabidiol on a regular schedule. If you're new to CBD, then microdosing is a great way to better understand the effects of CBD on your body and we suggest trying a microdosing schedule before beginning a full CBD regiment. This helps you find a sweet-spot dose that works best for your body. Microdosing is also great for people experienced with CBD that want to reset their system and get back into their optimal therapeutic range, as we can develop a tolerance over time. Microdosing involves taking very low doses of a substance, usually a psychedelic drug. The amount of the substance that is used is significantly below a hallucinogenic dose, yet proponents believe that the practice can produce a range of positive health effects.

These low doses are purported to enhance daily functioning while avoiding a dramatically altered state of consciousness.

People are motivated to microdose for a number of reasons. These include a desire to:

Alleviate mental health symptoms (such as anxiety and depression)

Enhance performance

Facilitate social interactions

Improve creativity

Increased energy

Increase focus

Increase concentration

Reduce physical symptoms (such as muscle tension and headache)

Relieve from menstrual pain

Interest in microdosing has grown tremendously in recent years, spawning an abundance of online discussions, videos, and articles devoted to the practice. Despite the dramatic rise in prominence, research on the practice is still in its relative infancy.

Can microdosing really improve your mental health? Is it safe? Is it legal? The answer to those questions depends on various factors.

Little is known about the prevalence, effects, safety, and long-term impacts, so more research is needed to fully understand the potential help or harm that microdosing may hold. The legality of the practice depends on the substances used—two of the most popular substances are illegal, but some others can be legally microdosed.

History of Microdosing

Psychedelics are powerful psychoactive substances that produce mind-altering effects including changes in perception, mood, and cognition.1
Early research on the use of psychedelics showed a number of beneficial effects.2 Psychiatrists used psychedelics during experiments during the 1940s, 1950s, and 1960s. It was during the 1960s that counterculture figures such as psychologist Timothy Leary helped to popularize hallucinogens. However, research on the topic was effectively halted for a period of 40 years after such substances were banned in the United States. The practice of microdosing has grown considerably in recent years, particularly as it has gotten media coverage from a number of high profile publications. Interest in microdosing has grown alongside related practices such as the use of "smart drugs" and nootropics.

Substances

Definitions of what exactly constitutes a microdose vary. Generally, it involves taking about 5% to 10% of a recreational dose of a hallucinogenic substance. This amounts to somewhere between 10 and 20 micrograms. Substances that are often used for microdosing include:

Ayahuasca

This psychoactive brew or tea originates in South American that is used as part of some religious ceremonies.

Cannabidiol (CBD)

CBD is the second most abundant cannabinoid found in marijuana. It is non-psychoactive and is believed to help relieve anxiety and stress.

Cannabis

Also known as marijuana, it may also be used to microdose and is purported to help relieve anxiety and improve focus.

Ibogaine

This is a root bark cultivated in Central Africa and sometimes used in traditional spiritual medicine. Some research suggests it may hold promise for relieving opioid dependence.

Ketamine

This medication is usually used for inducing and maintaining pain relief and sedation during surgery.

Lysergic acid diethylamide (LSD)

LSD is considered the most popular substance for microdosing, it is said to help people feel more focused, productive, and creative.

Mescaline (peyote)

Mescaline is a naturally-occurring psychedelic that has effects similar to LSD and has played an important role in Native American tradition. While illegal in the U.S., its use is legal for certain religious groups and for scientific research.

Methylenedioxyamphetamine (MDMA)

Popularly known as ecstasy or molly, MDMA is a psychoactive drug that is primarily used for recreational purposes. It has energizing effects and enhances feelings of empathy and self-awareness.

Methylphenidate (Ritalin)

This medication is used to treat ADHD and narcolepsy, but is sometimes used recreationally to enhance academic or athletic performance.

Nicotine

Popularly consumed in tobacco products, people who microdose nicotine suggest that it can help improve memory and focus.

N,N-dimethyltryptamine (DMT)

DMT produces short but intense psychedelic experiences. When microdosed, proponents suggest that it helps increase spiritual awareness and lessen feelings of anxiety.

Psilocybin ("magic" mushrooms)

Like LSD, psilocybin one of the most popular substances used in microdosing. Some research suggests that the substance may have antidepressant effects.5
While a number of different substances can be used, those most commonly utilized for microdosing are the psychedelics LSD and psilocybin. These tend to be the most researched and are often easier to obtain than some lesser-used substances.
It is important to note that LSD, psilocybin, ibogaine, and DMT are all classified as Schedule I drugs by the Drug Enforcement Administration (DEA), which means that their possession, use, and distribution is illegal in the United States.

Effects

There is a lack of research into the effects and potential benefits of microdosing. Another problem is that researchers do not yet know the possible long-term effects of this practice. Of the research that has been done so far, most of these studies rely on respondents self-reporting their past experiences with microdosing. Such studies may not give a full depiction of the practice, since most of these participants already expect to have a good experience so their feedback may be biased. In order to determine if microdosing has the potential to improve mental well-being or treat certain mental disorders, there needs to be randomized controlled trials that compare the effects of microdosing to that of placebo.

Perceived Benefits

In one study asking about perceived benefits, participants reported the following positive outcomes:
Improved mood
Improved focus
Creativity
Self-efficacy
Increased energy
Social benefits
Cognitive benefits
Reduced anxiety
Creativity

Increased creativity is one of the most commonly reported benefits of microdosing, but it is also one of the most difficult to measure. People might feel that they are more creative, but this may not necessarily correspond to real-world improvements in problem-solving and innovation. While further investigation is needed, respondents do report feeling more focused, mindful, and engaged with the world around them. Greater openness, curiosity, shifting perspectives, and overall greater feelings of creativity are commonly reported benefits.

Mental Health

People who report microdosing often do so in order to help alleviate the symptoms of stress, anxiety, or depression. One study found that mental health was one of the key reasons why many people decided to try microdosing, and 44% of participants reported that the practice led to improvements in their mental health.6 Another study published in the journal Frontiers in Psychiatry asked participants via an online questionnaire about their experiences with microdosing. The participants in the study were over the age of 18 and had been diagnosed with at least one mental health condition. The results suggested that many participants felt that microdosing was more effective than some other types of conventional treatment, yet not as effective as standard doses of psychedelics.7

Well-Being

People frequently report feelings of improvements in mood such as greater happiness, peace, calm, well-being, reduced depressive symptoms, optimism, and a better outlook on life. Cognitive and social benefits are also commonly reported. These include such things as improved mental clarity, greater empathy, and higher levels of extraversion. People who have tried microdosing also commonly report experiencing a range of other perceived benefits including the general lack of side effects, the ability to control the dose, and the novelty of the experience itself.7

Full-Dose vs. Microdose

While there is still a lack of research on microdosing, some recent evidence suggests that full-dose psychedelics may have some benefits. Despite earlier concerns, research has found no link between the use of psychedelics and later mental illness or suicidal actions.8 In fact, in some reports, these substances were associated with a lower rate of mental health issues.

Some studies have found that LSD and psilocybin may be useful in the treatment of drug and alcohol dependence10 and depression.11 Also, MDMA has shown some benefits in the treatment of post-traumatic stress disorder (PTSD).12

Psychedelics have been shown to increase openness. Some research suggests that psychedelics (at full doses) may help relieve some mental health conditions including anxiety and depression. What might this suggest in terms of microdosing? It is important to remember that while these substances have been shown in some studies to have therapeutic potential at full doses, this does not necessarily mean that people will experience the same effects at sub-hallucinogenic doses.

Microdosing offers some advantages over the use of full-dose psychedelics. While these substances tend to have low physiological risks, full doses do place people at the risk of experiencing psychological side effects including what is popularly referred as having a "bad trip."

A "bad trip" is an experience characterized by frightening hallucinations, paranoia, mood swings, and delusions that can potentially be dangerous. So while standard doses of psychedelics appear to offer some benefits, they are not always desirable due to the alterations in perceptions, cognitions, and emotions as well as the potential for unwanted side effects.

Because microdosing involves much lower doses, people are less likely to have these negative side effects. However, it is also important to be aware that even sub-hallucinogenic doses of these substances can produce unwanted and unpleasant side effects.

Because of the promising potential seen in research on standard doses of psychedelic substances, the potential of microdosing as a mental health and substance use treatment warrants further research.

Safety and Risks

Microdosing may provide some benefits to some people, but that does not mean that it is without unwanted effects. In one study, participants reported a number of challenges associated with microdosing. Some reported problems included:

Physiological discomfort
Impaired focus
Impaired energy
Increased symptoms
Impaired mood
Increased anxiety
Social interference
Cognitive interference

Some people with certain medical conditions such as anxiety may find that these substances can make their symptoms worse. People who have a history of psychotic disorders such as schizophrenia or bipolar disorder may want to also avoid psychedelic substances at any dosage level.

Another important safety consideration is the fact that because many of the substances used for microdosing are illegal, there is no regulation of the manufacture and production of these substances. One study found that MDMA tablets are often mixed with other substances including bath salts and only 60% of these tablets even contained any MDMA at all. This means that when you obtain these substances, it is very difficult to know what you are actually getting.

Legality

The most commonly reported challenge for people who have tried microdosing is the fact that these substances are illegal. For example, LSD, psilocybin, and peyote are all listed as Schedule I drugs in the Controlled Substances Act. The Drug Enforcement Administration (DEA) describes these substances as having "no currently accepted medical use and a high potential for abuse."[14] This means that it is illegal to cultivate, possess, or sell such substances for either personal use or distribution.

Such substances may also show up on standard drug tests, even at very low doses. This could lead to serious consequences, including legal charges and loss of employment.

Professional Considerations

Psychedelic-assisted therapy refers to any type of therapeutic practice that is assisted with the ingestion of a psychedelic drug. While research on this practice was largely halted after the passage of the Controlled Substances Act, there has been a recent resurgence in interest in the clinical use of psychedelics as part of therapeutic treatment. It is important to note that these substances are still illegal and cannot be legally prescribed or given by a doctor or psychiatrist. However, as more research is done on the use of psychedelics, both in standard dosages and microdoses, it may be possible that psychedelics find their way into various treatment paradigms.[15] There has been a recent push to reclassify psychedelics as Schedule II controlled substances.[16] This would recognize that these have medical uses, which would make it possible to conduct further research and utilize them in clinical, supervised settings. Whether this happens, however, remains to be seen.

What Does CBD Feel Like?

Cannabidiol, or short for CBD, is one of the 113 known compounds called cannabinoids found in the Cannabis sativa L. plant, also known as simply hemp. CBD is known to support the mind and body in many wonderful ways. Among the many benefits that users notice and see results from, some of the main benefits of CBD are a sense of calm & relaxation, supports healthy sleep cycles, helps in recovery from exercise-induced inflammation, and more. So what does CBD feel like when you take it? Does CBD oil relax you? Does CBD make you feel good? Does CBD oil give you a buzz? We'll get into that, but first, it's important to note something.
It mostly depends on what your body needs.
CBD acts as an adaptogenic, also referred to as "adaptogens," which is "defined as agents that support the body's ability to accommodate varying physical and emotional stresses" to influence more of what your body needs while promoting overall health and wellness.

The Human Endocannabinoid System

Before getting into how does CBD feel, it's important we cover what the Endocannabinoid System is. What CBD feels like happens when it interacts with our Endocannabinoid System
CBD works by activating the Endocannabinoid System, or ECS, indirectly by a channel of receptors within our central and peripheral nervous system located in our brain, spinal cord, organs, and immune system.
Cannabinoids behave differently, so one might trigger only one receptor, while others bind with both. In some cases, like CBD, the cannabinoids don't bind to CB1 or CB2, instead, altering those receptors through other pathways.
Cannabinoids act as a primer for nerve endings, allowing your brain to communicate more effectively with your body. The goal of this to get your body back to normal healthy levels or equilibrium called "homeostasis." This explains why taking CBD doesn't necessarily bring immediate results, but consumers see the real benefits of CBD over time of consistent use.

What Does CBD Feel Like? Can You Feel CBD?

Unlike many natural remedies, CBD does have an effect that on yourself that you will feel. When you take CBD, it takes about 15-45 minutes to feel an effect. Keep in mind that CBD is not like THC, where you feel "high," but you feel a subtle effect of calm and relaxation. When you talk about CBD's ability to help mitigate symptoms of anxiety, pain, inflammation, and other health cases, it can take a couple of days, 3 to 7 days, to 2-4 weeks of consistent dosing to notice results.

That depends more on how bad your case is, your body's response and tolerance to CBD, the quality of the CBD product, and your individual biology.

So how does CBD make you feel? It depends on a few things.

What's impressive – and perplexing – is CBD's versatility. To better understand this, let's have to look at CBD's potential adaptogenic properties.

Adaptogens are plants or extracts that help the body adapt to stresses and biological changes, including immune system activity. Theoretically, both Cannabis sativa L. and full-spectrum whole-plant extract could fit the adaptogen definition. However, CBD itself is a molecule – not a plant or extract.

But labels aside, CBD products display the same behaviors you'll see from verified adaptogens.

Thanks to its adaptogenic performance, CBD extracts' effects differ – even contradict – depending on your body's needs. For instance, your brain will be more active during the day, so you may notice a clearer head and more energy. The opposite will be true at night, with many people using CBD as a sleep aid or for general relaxation during inactive periods. Another example is CBD's seemingly opposing impact on eating habits. One 2018 CBD study noted both increased and decreased appetite as a side effect, depending on which participant they examined. Overall, CBD can be either relaxing or stimulating, depending on what your brain and body need. Regardless, you won't notice any physical or mental impairment like THC produces.

How Does CBD Make You Feel If You Take High Doses?

If you think higher doses mean better effects, you're not alone. After all, it makes perfect sense. But we should know by now that CBD seems to defy conventional expectations. CBD behaves in a "bell curve" or "u-shaped" fashion when it comes to dosing. Its effects are biphasic, meaning there's a negative correlation between dose and potency – as dose increases, effectiveness eventually decreases.

CBD & Cannabinoids Biphasic Explained Graph on how Cannabinoids have diminishing effects at higher doses

In other words, too much CBD is just as ineffective as too little. Dosage requirements can range from tens to hundreds of milligrams per day. But if you exceed the "sweet spot" dose, the effects will weaken and eventually stop.

Another problem is that taking higher doses can cause tolerance, forcing you to take a three to seven-day CBD break and get back on a lower dose to allow your tolerance to CBD to reset. However, CBD is known to have side effects, which will intensify as you increase the dose. We'll get to that in a minute.

Does CBD Oil Give You A Buzz or High?

No, CBD oil won't give you a buzz or high feeling. THC and – to a much lesser extent – cannabinol (CBN) are the only two major cannabinoids known to impair mental and motor function. As we mentioned, CBD doesn't bind to the CB1 or CB2 receptors, meaning it can't directly affect the way THC and many other cannabinoids do. Instead, cannabidiol works through different pathways, altering the shape and behavior of endocannabinoid receptors.
Once altered, the CB1 and CB2 receptors may bind differently – or not at all – to other cannabinoids. For instance, not only will CBD not get you as high, but its effects block the uptake of THC, meaning cannabidiol can mitigate and shorten THC intoxication.

Microdosing CBD for Beginners

Is Microdosing a Long term Solution?

It's important to note that microdosing isn't always the most effective way to ingest CBD products to gain the full therapeutic effects, but it can be! It's a great way to discover your right amount of measurable cannabidiol dosage over the course of a couple of days. After you've found the amount that works for you, then you can begin to take that amount once or twice per day, and continue increasing as needed.

Microdosing with CBD Tinctures

CBD tinctures are typically packaged in 15-mL or 30-mL bottles and each bottle varies in terms of concentration and effects, ranging in CBD concentration from 100mg to 5000mg per bottle.

*First thing to note, there are TWO measurements happening: the liquid ML measurement of the oil, and the MG measurement of the CBD concentration within that liquid.

The key to understanding tincture dosing is noting the serving size, which is typically 1ml of oil, or one full dropper. However, many times it is .25ml or .5ml (a quarter or half of the dropper) so it's important to read the labels! (If you're new to CBD and are overwhelmed already, chat with our Budtenders about finding a low concentrated product to start with.)

To find the strength per serving, divide the total mg-strength of a bottle by the total number of servings. A 1000mg strength tincture in a 30-mL bottle features 30 1-mL servings of roughly 33.3mg of CBD. Luckily, most tincture droppers feature dosage measurements that make it easy for the consumer to take the right amount so just make sure to read your labels.

To microdose a tincture, it's important to find out how many drops are in one mL of oil to determine the strength of each drop. As an example, if your dropper has 24 drops in a 1 mL serving, and each dropper full is 33mg of CBD, then one drop comes out to just about 1.4mg of CBD per drop. So, instead of taking one full dropper of 33mg of CBD at one time, instead, you ingest 2mg of CBD every hour or two to gradually feel the effects and find out the right amount for your body.

*For beginners, we suggest starting with a dose of < 5mg-10mg of CBD. You may notice subtle drowsiness and muscle relaxation. Pay attention to your body and your mind. The more you ingest, the more sleepy you may feel, so make sure to not operate a vehicle or heavy machinery.

Microdosing Cbd Edibles

Tinctures are just one method for consuming CBD. They are a great place to start because you can tailor the dose to your personal needs. However, there are many other low-dose products on the market such as mints, capsules, tablets, and even delicious treats like chocolates and gummies! Chat with our team to learn what's best for you and the issue you are treating.

Create a Microdosing Schedule

Below is an example of how to begin your new microdosing schedule, but remember that every body is different, so listen to your body and intuition when working with the plant. When it comes to CBD tinctures, begin with one micro-serving of CBD in hour one. After one hour has passed, take two drops of CBD oil. After the second hour has passed, take three drops of CBD oil. Continue this process until you can begin to feel the effects of your CBD oil. After you've found your sweet spot, add up the totals to discover the right measurement of CBD oil that works for your body.

8 am – 1 drop of CBD oil
9 am – 2 drops of CBD oil
10 am – 3 drops of CBD oil
11 am – 4 drops of CBD oil
12 pm – 5 drop of CBD oil.

After one morning of microdosing, you'll have taken just over one half of a full dropper of CBD tincture. If you don't feel any therapeutic effects, then continue to add drops to your schedule every hour until you've established the therapeutic range that works for you.

Build a Microdosing Journal

Before you begin your new microdosing regiment, it's important to outline a schedule and give yourself a chance to take notes on how you feel after each drop of CBD oil. After you take each microdose, answer these questions in a simple notebook:

CBD Dark Chocolate by Kiva Confections
CBD Dark Chocolate by Kiva Confections
1 – What is my pain level on a scale of 1-10?
2 – How comfortable and calm am I?
3 – Am I feeling better than before I began microdosing?
4 – Is it easy to breathe?
5 – On a scale of 1 – 10, how relaxed do I feel?

By answering these questions at different dosage intervals, you can begin to track your progress and identify the therapeutic range of CBD dosage that works for you.

Find CBD Products at Mission Cannabis Club

MCC has a wide variety of CBD products that are perfect for CBD enthusiasts of all experience levels. Checkout our menu to learn about our CBD edibles, oils, vape cartridges and other CBD goods to find the right product that works for you.

Microdosing And Me: A Useful (And Honest) Guide To CBD And Pain

Up to 8 million people live with life-altering chronic pain in the UK. For Niamh O'Donoghue, whose own health journey saw her undergo multiple aggressive spine-correcting surgeries, kidney failure and a destructive cancer diagnosis – all before the age of 25 – CBD offered relief when she needed it most.

One of my earliest memories is of pain. My teenage years were filled with hospital appointments, calendars circled with dates for surgery. At 13, over the course of one night, my spine twisted like a plumbing trap to more than 80 degrees. At one point, a piece of hardware from the titanium rods supporting my spine pierced through my skin. It was like a bomb going off in my bones.

Later, a pain-induced blackout on a beach with friends resulted in kidney failure. Then, there were the menstrual cramps and chronic fatigue. Later still, a suspicious lump on my thyroid gland that turned out to be cancerous resulted in surgery from ear-to-ear – like a permanent smiley face on my neck – and a heavy blast of radiation. Over the last 27 years my body has been rendered useless and immobile. I know what it feels like to hit peak on the pain-o-meter.

In a bid to regain some autonomy over my pain – and to rid my body of years of toxins – I've spent the last few years seeking out alternative pain management treatments. I've tried reiki sessions and mindfulness, pilates and swimming, non-medicated pain patches and hot water bottles. Then I found CBD (cannabidiol) oil. Not to be confused with medical cannabis, CBD is made from hemp, a variety of the cannabis plant which is low in the high-inducing THC. In the right dose and form, CBD really can help manage – not cure – a huge range of health issues, including chronic pain.

"It's probably a little bit of a false claim to say that CBD is a sole cure for chronic pain," says scientific advisor to The Drug Store Dr Julie Moltke, whose book A Quick Guide To CBD was published in June and is a practical guide for anyone interested in learning more about CBD. Studies show that CBD interacts with our endocannabinoid system – the body's own anti-depressant – to restore balance and reduce inflammation, and so if you take it in high enough doses you get an "anti-inflammatory effect throughout the whole body", explains Dr Moltke. "It can also be used for endometriosis… and it's even been medically proven to help the symptoms of epilepsy," she continues.

CBD won't mend a broken bone, it won't fix my crooked spine. But for some, it's the holy grail of anxiety solutions. And for others, like me, it can offer a brief moment of respite from the sting of sciatica, or the dull ache of period pains.

Here, a guide to using CBD to treat pain effectively – with the caveat that one should always seek advice from a medical professional.

The A To Z Of CBD

Not all CBD oils are created equal, nor do they perform in the same way. At present there are two camps of non-medicated CBD (meaning CBD without THC): full spectrum CBD and CBD isolate. Full spectrum is when the entirety of the hemp plant – stalk, seeds, roots leaves – is used to produce the final product. Cannabidiol is one of at least 140 different cannabinoids found in hemp plants, each with its own chemical properties, so with full spectrum CBD, the oil is mixed with other cannabinoids from within that plant. "That can often include a tiny bit of THC," says Olivia Ferdi, co-founder of Trip. "In theory, it means you're getting the benefit of other cannabinoids working in tandem with the CBD in different ways that aren't necessarily fully understood yet, but studies suggest they have positive effects."
On the other end of the spectrum is isolate CBD, which is where only the CBD cannabinoids have been extracted. In essence, it's a more refined version of CBD and is beneficial for those who want to measure their full intake of CBD.
Ferdi, whose millennial pink bottle of 300mg orange blossom CBD was among the first I tried during lockdown and is great for CBD newcomers, compares the two ends of the CBD spectrum to eating an orange versus taking a vitamin C tablet: "We know a vitamin C tablet will do a great job and you're going to absorb it well but, maybe the orange is better for you because of the fibres and fruit sugars it contains."
Broad spectrum CBD, then, falls in the middle of both isolate and full spectrum CBD. Neither camp has been proven to be right or wrong.
"Medicinal cannabis is very good at decreasing pain that's coming from the central nervous system," Dr Moltke tells me of her experience of treating chronic pain patients with CBD and THC (the principal psychoactive component of cannabis). "We know for a fact the endocannabinoid regulates pain and pain perception. When we use the whole plant, you can decrease pain – especially chronic pain, also called neuropathic pain."

Find The Right Brand For You

From chewing gum to bath bombs, balms to serums, there is truly a wealth of CBD products to choose from (the CBD market is set to reach $1.8 billion by 2022, up from half a billion in 2018). I first tried oral oil because it has a faster absorption rate. Trip's selection appealed to me because of the natural flavours (elderflower mint, peach ginger, lemon basil), and the oils proved calming and tasted pleasant. The very process of taking CBD oil is, in itself, a form of self-care. It's important to let the oil sit under your tongue rather than haphazardly chucking it back, as Ferdi explains: "Holding an oil in your mouth for 60 seconds – whether you realise it or not you've basically just created a self-care ritual. It's so hard to not talk in that one minute! It's a moment of stillness."

Celtic Winds medium strength 5 per cent CBD oil is a good middle-of-the-road option, if you can get past the earthy taste. A small amount of Greenheart's Full Spectrum Hemp Homogenised Oil goes a long way, and was effective for defusing a muscle spasm in my back when used in conjunction with over-the-counter pain relief.

Pollen's Powerbank CBD Gummies didn't prove particularly fruitful for my stiff joints, but provided a little midday pep and curbed my workday stress (chewing distracts one's mind from Zoom). The limoncello packaging brightened my desk, too.

The Ohana skincare range combines gentle and caring skincare ingredients with the soothing benefits of CBD. When applied to the face with a cold jade roller or Gua Sha stone, I found the All-In-One Wonder Balm to be a welcome bedtime rescue. Similarly, Oto's rosemary and peppermint Focus Roll-On provided targeted light relief, and the scent made me feel grounded.

"It's about finding a consistent source that's good quality," remarks Ferdi, whose premium brand Trip has witnessed a 420 per cent increase in sales since strict social distancing was introduced. Ferdi's advice rings particularly true when you consider that more than half of the most popular CBD oils sold in pharmacies, health stores and online have been found not to contain the level of CBD promised on the label.

"In general, I would go for a broad spectrum product: a product which contains all the different cannabinoids," Dr Moltke says. "It's worth trying a reliable brand. If they do have good delivery methods, that's a plus."

Keep A Pain Journal

To echo Dr Moltke, CBD is not the final solution to pain management, but can greatly reduce inflammation and reduce muscle fatigue – and yes, it helped soothe my quarantine aches and pains, too. Building CBD into my daily schedule allowed me to become more mindful of my body, and to take heed of when it needed rest. A daily pain journal helped me to distinguish the niggles from the serious spasms, menstrual cramps from a leaky gut. I learned to listen to signals and know when CBD alone would be enough, versus when back-up was required.

Overall, there is a startling absence of information online when it comes to exact CBD dosing recommendations, but through research I've learned that a reasonable and feasible dose of CBD is around 10-40 milligrams per day. My dose amounts ebb and flow until I feel I've reached my sweet spot.

A word on CBD and addiction: while it's possible to build a tolerance to CBD – similar to caffeine and sugar – it's not possible to overdose. Similarly, research suggests CBD doesn't cause any cognitive effects – unlike THC, where we know smoking cannabis can cause cognitive decline and memory impairment defects. As Dr Moltke explains: "This is not something we see with CBD. We do however need to get real long-term data. We don't have any consistent data on very long term effects, but as far as we know – and the World Health Organisation has echoed this – CBD is safe to use."

Find Your Community

My initial impulse to lump CBD in with other dubious "alternative" medicines was rooted in my own lack of knowledge and understanding. For beginners, Suzanne Gatt's easy listening podcast is informal but packed with information. Similarly, Dr Moltke's The Holistic Medicine Podcast debunks common myths, and delivers bite-sized snippets backed up by science and research.
And to the sceptics? When you've endured constant pain for a long time, you'll try anything after a while. CBD is, for me, a gentle elixir that helps extinguish the burn of nerve pain and lessens the churn of anxiety. And if it's good enough for Queen Victoria's menstrual cramps, then it's good enough for mine.

7 Benefits and Uses of CBD Oil (Plus Side Effects)

Cannabidiol is a popular natural remedy used for many common ailments. Better known as CBD, it is one of over 100 chemical compounds known as cannabinoids found in the cannabis or marijuana plant, Cannabis sativa.
Tetrahydrocannabinol (THC) is the main psychoactive cannabinoid found in cannabis, and causes the sensation of getting "high" that's often associated with marijuana. However, unlike THC, CBD is not psychoactive.
This quality makes CBD an appealing option for those who are looking for relief from pain and other symptoms without the mind-altering effects of marijuana or certain pharmaceutical drugs.
CBD oil is made by extracting CBD from the cannabis plant, then diluting it with a carrier oil like coconut or hemp seed oil. It's gaining momentum in the health and wellness world, with some scientific studies confirming it may ease symptoms of ailments like chronic pain and anxiety.
Here are seven health benefits of CBD oil that are backed by scientific evidence.

1. Can Relieve Pain

Marijuana has been used to treat pain as far back as 2900 B.C. More recently, scientists have discovered that certain components of marijuana, including CBD, are responsible for its pain-relieving effects. The human body contains a specialized system called the endocannabinoid system (ECS), which is involved in regulating a variety of functions including sleep, appetite, pain and immune system response. The body produces endocannabinoids, which are neurotransmitters that bind to cannabinoid receptors in your nervous system. Studies have shown that CBD may help reduce chronic pain by impacting endocannabinoid receptor activity, reducing inflammation and interacting with neurotransmitters.

For example, one study in rats found that CBD injections reduced pain response to surgical incision, while another rat study found that oral CBD treatment significantly reduced sciatic nerve pain and inflammation. Several human studies have found that a combination of CBD and THC is effective in treating pain related to multiple sclerosis and arthritis. An oral spray called Sativex, which is a combination of THC and CBD, is approved in several countries to treat pain related to multiple sclerosis. One study of 47 people with multiple sclerosis examined the effects of taking Sativex for one month. The participants experienced improvements in pain, walking, and muscle spasms. Still, the study didn't include any control group and placebo effects cannot be ruled out. Another study found that Sativex significantly improved pain during movement, pain at rest and sleep quality in 58 people with rheumatoid arthritis (8Trusted Source).

2. Could Reduce Anxiety and Depression

Anxiety and depression are common mental health disorders that can have devastating impacts on health and well-being. According to the World Health Organization, depression is the single largest contributor to disability worldwide, while anxiety disorders are ranked sixth. Anxiety and depression are usually treated with pharmaceutical drugs, which can cause a number of side effects including drowsiness, agitation, insomnia, sexual dysfunction and headache (10Trusted Source). What's more, medications like benzodiazepines can be addictive and may lead to substance abuse. CBD oil has shown promise as a treatment for both depression and anxiety, leading many who live with these disorders to become interested in this natural approach. In one Brazilian study, 57 men received either oral CBD or a placebo 90 minutes before they underwent a simulated public speaking test. The researchers found that a 300-mg dose of CBD was the most effective at significantly reducing anxiety during the test.
The placebo, a 150-mg dose of CBD, and a 600-mg dose of CBD had little to no effect on anxiety. CBD oil has even been used to safely treat insomnia and anxiety in children with post-traumatic stress disorder. CBD has also shown antidepressant-like effects in several animal studies. These qualities are linked to CBD's ability to act on the brain's receptors for serotonin, a neurotransmitter that regulates mood and social behavior.

3. Can Alleviate Cancer-Related Symptoms

CBD may help reduce symptoms related to cancer and side effects related to cancer treatment, like nausea, vomiting and pain. One study looked at the effects of CBD and THC in 177 people with cancer-related pain who did not experience relief from pain medication. Those treated with an extract containing both compounds experienced a significant reduction in pain compared to those who received only THC extract. CBD may also help reduce chemotherapy-induced nausea and vomiting, which are among the most common chemotherapy-related side effects for those with cancer. Though there are drugs that help with these distressing symptoms, they are sometimes ineffective, leading some people to seek alternatives. A study of 16 people undergoing chemotherapy found that a one-to-one combination of CBD and THC administered via mouth spray reduced chemotherapy-related nausea and vomiting better than standard treatment alone. Some test-tube and animal studies have even shown that CBD may have anticancer properties. For example, one test-tube study found that concentrated CBD induced cell death in human breast cancer cells. Another study showed that CBD inhibited the spread of aggressive breast cancer cells in mice. However, these are test-tube and animal studies, so they can only suggest what might work in people. More studies in humans are needed before conclusions can be made.

4. May Reduce Acne

Acne is a common skin condition that affects more than 9% of the population. It is thought to be caused by a number of factors, including genetics, bacteria, underlying inflammation and the overproduction of sebum, an oily secretion made by sebaceous glands in the skin. Based on recent scientific studies, CBD oil may help treat acne due to its anti-inflammatory properties and ability to reduce sebum production. One test-tube study found that CBD oil prevented sebaceous gland cells from secreting excessive sebum, exerted anti-inflammatory actions and prevented the activation of "pro-acne" agents like inflammatory cytokines. Another study had similar findings, concluding that CBD may be an efficient and safe way to treat acne, thanks in part to its remarkable anti-inflammatory qualities. Though these results are promising, human studies exploring the effects of CBD on acne are needed.

5. Might Have Neuroprotective Properties

Researchers believe that CBD's ability to act on the endocannabinoid system and other brain signaling systems may provide benefits for those with neurological disorders. In fact, one of the most studied uses for CBD is in treating neurological disorders like epilepsy and multiple sclerosis. Though research in this area is still relatively new, several studies have shown promising results. Sativex, an oral spray consisting of CBD and THC, has been proven to be a safe and effective way to reduce muscle spasticity in people with multiple sclerosis. One study found that Sativex reduced spasms in 75% of 276 people with multiple sclerosis who were experiencing muscle spasticity that was resistant to medication. Another study gave 214 people with severe epilepsy 0.9–2.3 grams of CBD oil per pound (2–5 g/kg) of body weight. Their seizures reduced by a median of 36.5%. One more study found that CBD oil significantly reduced seizure activity in children with Dravet syndrome, a complex childhood epilepsy disorder, compared to a placebo. However, it's important to note that some people in both these studies experienced adverse reactions associated with CBD treatment, such as convulsions, fever and fatigue.

CBD has also been researched for its potential effectiveness in treating several other neurological diseases. For example, several studies have shown that treatment with CBD improved quality of life and sleep quality for people with Parkinson's disease. Additionally, animal and test-tube studies have shown that CBD may decrease inflammation and help prevent the neurodegeneration associated with Alzheimer's disease. In one long-term study, researchers gave CBD to mice genetically predisposed to Alzheimer's disease, finding that it helped prevent cognitive decline

6. Could Benefit Heart Health

Recent research has linked CBD with several benefits for the heart and circulatory system, including the ability to lower high blood pressure. High blood pressure is linked to higher risks of a number of health conditions, including stroke, heart attack and metabolic syndroms. Studies indicate that CBD may be able to help with high blood pressure.

One recent study treated nine healthy men with one dose of 600 mg of CBD oil and found it reduced resting blood pressure, compared to a placebo. The same study also gave the men stress tests that normally increase blood pressure. Interestingly, the single dose of CBD led the men to experience a smaller blood pressure increase than normal in response to these tests. Researchers have suggested that the stress- and anxiety-reducing properties of CBD are responsible for its ability to help lower blood pressure. Additionally, several animal studies have demonstrated that CBD may help reduce the inflammation and cell death associated with heart disease due to its powerful antioxidant and stress-reducing properties. For example, one study found that treatment with CBD reduced oxidative stress and prevented heart damage in diabetic mice with heart disease.

7. Several Other Potential Benefits

CBD has been studied for its role in treating a number of health issues other than those outlined above. Though more studies are needed, CBD is thought to provide the following health benefits:

Antipsychotic effects: Studies suggest that CBD may help people with schizophrenia and other mental disorders by reducing psychotic symptoms.

Substance abuse treatment: CBD has been shown to modify circuits in the brain related to drug addiction. In rats, CBD has been shown to reduce morphine dependence and heroin-seeking behavior.

Anti-tumor effects: In test-tube and animal studies, CBD has demonstrated anti-tumor effects. In animals, it has been shown to prevent the spread of breast, prostate, brain, colon and lung cancer.

Diabetes prevention: In diabetic mice, treatment with CBD reduced the incidence of diabetes by 56% and significantly reduced inflammation.

Summary Some studies suggest that CBD may help with diabetes, substance abuse, mental disorders and certain types of cancers. However, more research in humans is needed.

Are There Any Side Effects?

Though CBD is generally well tolerated and considered safe, it may cause adverse reactions in some people.

Side effects noted in studies include:

Diarrhea

Changes in appetite and weight

Fatigue

CBD is also known to interact with several medications. Before you start using CBD oil, discuss it with your doctor to ensure your safety and avoid potentially harmful interactions. This is especially important if you take medications or supplements that come with a "grapefruit warning." Both grapefruit and CBD interfere with cytochromes P450 (CYPs), a group of enzymes that are important to drug metabolism. One study performed on mice showed that CBD-rich cannabis extracts have the potential to cause liver toxicity. However, some the mice in the study were force-fed extremely large doses of the extract

www.ingramcontent.com/pod-product-compliance
Lightning Source LLC
LaVergne TN
LVHW081517060526
838200LV00005B/197